Cycle Track

Month:__________

Sunday	Monday	Tuesday	Wednesday	Thursday	Friday	Saturday

Cycle Tracker

Month:__________

Sunday	Monday	Tuesday	Wednesday	Thursday	Friday	Saturday

Cycle Tracker

Month: ___________

Sunday	Monday	Tuesday	Wednesday	Thursday	Friday	Saturday

Cycle Tracker

Month:___________

Sunday	Monday	Tuesday	Wednesday	Thursday	Friday	Saturday

Cycle Tracker

Month:____________

Sunday	Monday	Tuesday	Wednesday	Thursday	Friday	Saturday

Cycle Tracker

Month:___________

Sunday	Monday	Tuesday	Wednesday	Thursday	Friday	Saturday

Cycle Tracker

Month:__________

Sunday	Monday	Tuesday	Wednesday	Thursday	Friday	Saturday

Cycle Tracker

Month:__________

Sunday	Monday	Tuesday	Wednesday	Thursday	Friday	Saturday

Cycle Tracker

Month:__________

Sunday	Monday	Tuesday	Wednesday	Thursday	Friday	Saturday

Cycle Tracker

Month: ____________

Sunday	Monday	Tuesday	Wednesday	Thursday	Friday	Saturday

Cycle Tracker

Month: ___________

Sunday	Monday	Tuesday	Wednesday	Thursday	Friday	Saturday

Appointments

Date	Time	Doctor	Questions	Notes
9/8/2020	3:00 pm			
9/30/2020	3:00pm	Nurse Hailey		

Appointments

Date	Time	Doctor	Questions	Notes

Retrieval Medications

Medication	Dose																															

Medication	Dose																															

NOTES & REMINDERS

Retrieval Results

Retrieved	
Fertilized	
Day 3	
Day 5	
Made to freeze!	

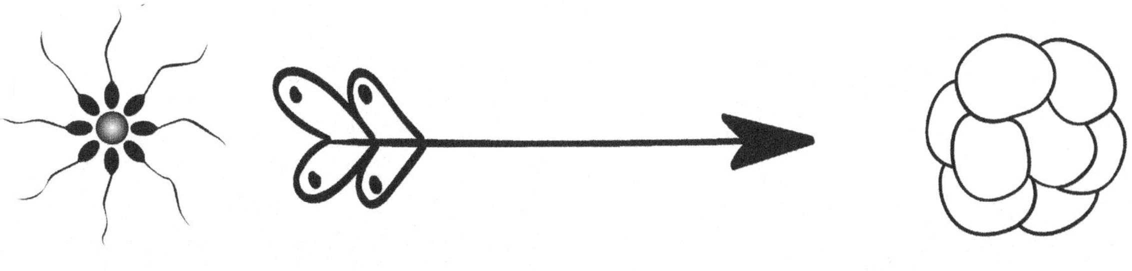

Transfer Medications

Medication	Dose

Medication	Dose

NOTES & REMINDERS

My Week at a Glance

Week of:____________________

MY WEEKLY AGENDA: NOTES

Sunday ....

Monday ....

Tuesday ....

Wednesday ....

Thursday ....

Friday ....

Saturday ....

TOP GOALS

TOP TO DO OF THE WEEK

HEALTHY EATING TRACKER

M	T	W	T	F	S	S

QUOTE OF THE DAY

TODAY I AM GRATEFUL FOR:

My Week at a Glance

Week of: ______________

MY WEEKLY AGENDA: NOTES

Sunday ....

Monday ....

Tuesday ....

Wednesday ....

Thursday ....

Friday ....

Saturday ....

TOP GOALS

TOP TO DO OF THE WEEK

HEALTHY EATING TRACKER

M	T	W	T	F	S	S
☐	☐	☐	☐	☐	☐	☐
☐	☐	☐	☐	☐	☐	☐
☐	☐	☐	☐	☐	☐	☐
☐	☐	☐	☐	☐	☐	☐
☐	☐	☐	☐	☐	☐	☐
☐	☐	☐	☐	☐	☐	☐
☐	☐	☐	☐	☐	☐	☐
☐	☐	☐	☐	☐	☐	☐

QUOTE OF THE DAY

TODAY I AM GRATEFUL FOR:

My Week at a Glance

Week of: ____________________

MY WEEKLY AGENDA: NOTES

Sunday ....

Monday ....

Tuesday ....

Wednesday ....

Thursday ....

Friday ....

Saturday ....

TOP GOALS

TOP TO DO OF THE WEEK

HEALTHY EATING TRACKER

M	T	W	T	F	S	S
☐	☐	☐	☐	☐	☐	☐
☐	☐	☐	☐	☐	☐	☐
☐	☐	☐	☐	☐	☐	☐
☐	☐	☐	☐	☐	☐	☐
☐	☐	☐	☐	☐	☐	☐
☐	☐	☐	☐	☐	☐	☐
☐	☐	☐	☐	☐	☐	☐
☐	☐	☐	☐	☐	☐	☐

QUOTE OF THE DAY

TODAY I AM GRATEFUL FOR:

My Week at a Glance

Week of: ____________________

MY WEEKLY AGENDA: NOTES

Sunday ....

Monday ....

Tuesday ....

Wednesday ....

Thursday ....

Friday ....

Saturday ....

TOP GOALS

TOP TO DO OF THE WEEK

HEALTHY EATING TRACKER

M	T	W	T	F	S	S
☐	☐	☐	☐	☐	☐	☐
☐	☐	☐	☐	☐	☐	☐
☐	☐	☐	☐	☐	☐	☐
☐	☐	☐	☐	☐	☐	☐
☐	☐	☐	☐	☐	☐	☐
☐	☐	☐	☐	☐	☐	☐
☐	☐	☐	☐	☐	☐	☐
☐	☐	☐	☐	☐	☐	☐

QUOTE OF THE DAY

TODAY I AM GRATEFUL FOR:

My Week at a Glance

Week of: ____________________

MY WEEKLY AGENDA: NOTES

Sunday ....

Monday ....

Tuesday ....

Wednesday ....

Thursday ....

Friday ....

Saturday ....

TOP GOALS

TOP TO DO OF THE WEEK

HEALTHY EATING TRACKER

M	T	W	T	F	S	S
☐	☐	☐	☐	☐	☐	☐
☐	☐	☐	☐	☐	☐	☐
☐	☐	☐	☐	☐	☐	☐
☐	☐	☐	☐	☐	☐	☐
☐	☐	☐	☐	☐	☐	☐
☐	☐	☐	☐	☐	☐	☐
☐	☐	☐	☐	☐	☐	☐
☐	☐	☐	☐	☐	☐	☐

QUOTE OF THE DAY

TODAY I AM GRATEFUL FOR:

My Week at a Glance

Week of: ____________________

MY WEEKLY AGENDA: NOTES

Sunday ....

Monday ....

Tuesday ....

Wednesday ....

Thursday ....

Friday ....

Saturday ....

TOP GOALS

TOP TO DO OF THE WEEK

HEALTHY EATING TRACKER

M	T	W	T	F	S	S
☐	☐	☐	☐	☐	☐	☐
☐	☐	☐	☐	☐	☐	☐
☐	☐	☐	☐	☐	☐	☐
☐	☐	☐	☐	☐	☐	☐
☐	☐	☐	☐	☐	☐	☐
☐	☐	☐	☐	☐	☐	☐
☐	☐	☐	☐	☐	☐	☐
☐	☐	☐	☐	☐	☐	☐

QUOTE OF THE DAY

TODAY I AM GRATEFUL FOR:

My Week at a Glance

Week of: ____________________

MY WEEKLY AGENDA: NOTES

Sunday ....

Monday ....

Tuesday ....

Wednesday ....

Thursday ....

Friday ....

Saturday ....

TOP GOALS

HEALTHY EATING TRACKER

M	T	W	T	F	S	S
☐	☐	☐	☐	☐	☐	☐
☐	☐	☐	☐	☐	☐	☐
☐	☐	☐	☐	☐	☐	☐
☐	☐	☐	☐	☐	☐	☐
☐	☐	☐	☐	☐	☐	☐
☐	☐	☐	☐	☐	☐	☐
☐	☐	☐	☐	☐	☐	☐
☐	☐	☐	☐	☐	☐	☐

TOP TO DO OF THE WEEK

QUOTE OF THE DAY

TODAY I AM GRATEFUL FOR:

My Week at a Glance

Week of: ____________________

MY WEEKLY AGENDA: NOTES

Sunday ....

Monday ....

Tuesday ....

Wednesday ....

Thursday ....

Friday ....

Saturday ....

TOP GOALS

HEALTHY EATING TRACKER

M	T	W	T	F	S	S
☐	☐	☐	☐	☐	☐	☐
☐	☐	☐	☐	☐	☐	☐
☐	☐	☐	☐	☐	☐	☐
☐	☐	☐	☐	☐	☐	☐
☐	☐	☐	☐	☐	☐	☐
☐	☐	☐	☐	☐	☐	☐
☐	☐	☐	☐	☐	☐	☐
☐	☐	☐	☐	☐	☐	☐

TOP TO DO OF THE WEEK

QUOTE OF THE DAY

TODAY I AM GRATEFUL FOR:

My Week at a Glance

Week of: ____________________

MY WEEKLY AGENDA: NOTES

Sunday ....

Monday ....

Tuesday ....

Wednesday ....

Thursday ....

Friday ....

Saturday ....

TOP GOALS

TOP TO DO OF THE WEEK

HEALTHY EATING TRACKER

M	T	W	T	F	S	S
☐	☐	☐	☐	☐	☐	☐
☐	☐	☐	☐	☐	☐	☐
☐	☐	☐	☐	☐	☐	☐
☐	☐	☐	☐	☐	☐	☐
☐	☐	☐	☐	☐	☐	☐
☐	☐	☐	☐	☐	☐	☐
☐	☐	☐	☐	☐	☐	☐
☐	☐	☐	☐	☐	☐	☐

QUOTE OF THE DAY

TODAY I AM GRATEFUL FOR:

My Week at a Glance

Week of: ____________________

MY WEEKLY AGENDA: NOTES

Sunday ....

Monday ....

Tuesday ....

Wednesday ....

Thursday ....

Friday ....

Saturday ....

TOP GOALS

HEALTHY EATING TRACKER

M	T	W	T	F	S	S
☐	☐	☐	☐	☐	☐	☐
☐	☐	☐	☐	☐	☐	☐
☐	☐	☐	☐	☐	☐	☐
☐	☐	☐	☐	☐	☐	☐
☐	☐	☐	☐	☐	☐	☐
☐	☐	☐	☐	☐	☐	☐
☐	☐	☐	☐	☐	☐	☐
☐	☐	☐	☐	☐	☐	☐

TOP TO DO OF THE WEEK

QUOTE OF THE DAY

TODAY I AM GRATEFUL FOR:

My Week at a Glance

Week of: ____________

MY WEEKLY AGENDA: NOTES

Sunday ....

Monday ....

Tuesday ....

Wednesday ....

Thursday ....

Friday ....

Saturday ....

TOP GOALS

HEALTHY EATING TRACKER

M	T	W	T	F	S	S
☐	☐	☐	☐	☐	☐	☐
☐	☐	☐	☐	☐	☐	☐
☐	☐	☐	☐	☐	☐	☐
☐	☐	☐	☐	☐	☐	☐
☐	☐	☐	☐	☐	☐	☐
☐	☐	☐	☐	☐	☐	☐
☐	☐	☐	☐	☐	☐	☐
☐	☐	☐	☐	☐	☐	☐

TOP TO DO OF THE WEEK

QUOTE OF THE DAY

TODAY I AM GRATEFUL FOR:

My Week at a Glance

Week of: ____________________

MY WEEKLY AGENDA: NOTES

Sunday ....

Monday ....

Tuesday ....

Wednesday ....

Thursday ....

Friday ....

Saturday ....

TOP GOALS

HEALTHY EATING TRACKER

M	T	W	T	F	S	S
☐	☐	☐	☐	☐	☐	☐
☐	☐	☐	☐	☐	☐	☐
☐	☐	☐	☐	☐	☐	☐
☐	☐	☐	☐	☐	☐	☐
☐	☐	☐	☐	☐	☐	☐
☐	☐	☐	☐	☐	☐	☐
☐	☐	☐	☐	☐	☐	☐
☐	☐	☐	☐	☐	☐	☐

TOP TO DO OF THE WEEK

QUOTE OF THE DAY

TODAY I AM GRATEFUL FOR:

My Week at a Glance

Week of: ____________________

MY WEEKLY AGENDA: NOTES

Sunday ....

Monday ....

Tuesday ....

Wednesday ....

Thursday ....

Friday ....

Saturday ....

TOP GOALS

TOP TO DO OF THE WEEK

HEALTHY EATING TRACKER

M	T	W	T	F	S	S
☐	☐	☐	☐	☐	☐	☐
☐	☐	☐	☐	☐	☐	☐
☐	☐	☐	☐	☐	☐	☐
☐	☐	☐	☐	☐	☐	☐
☐	☐	☐	☐	☐	☐	☐
☐	☐	☐	☐	☐	☐	☐
☐	☐	☐	☐	☐	☐	☐
☐	☐	☐	☐	☐	☐	☐

QUOTE OF THE DAY

TODAY I AM GRATEFUL FOR:

My Week at a Glance

Week of: ____________

MY WEEKLY AGENDA: NOTES

Sunday ....

Monday ....

Tuesday ....

Wednesday ....

Thursday ....

Friday ....

Saturday ....

TOP GOALS

TOP TO DO OF THE WEEK

HEALTHY EATING TRACKER

M	T	W	T	F	S	S
☐	☐	☐	☐	☐	☐	☐
☐	☐	☐	☐	☐	☐	☐
☐	☐	☐	☐	☐	☐	☐
☐	☐	☐	☐	☐	☐	☐
☐	☐	☐	☐	☐	☐	☐
☐	☐	☐	☐	☐	☐	☐
☐	☐	☐	☐	☐	☐	☐
☐	☐	☐	☐	☐	☐	☐

QUOTE OF THE DAY

TODAY I AM GRATEFUL FOR:

My Week at a Glance

Week of: ____________________

MY WEEKLY AGENDA: NOTES

Sunday ....

Monday ....

Tuesday ....

Wednesday ....

Thursday ....

Friday ....

Saturday ....

TOP GOALS

TOP TO DO OF THE WEEK

HEALTHY EATING TRACKER

M	T	W	T	F	S	S
☐	☐	☐	☐	☐	☐	☐
☐	☐	☐	☐	☐	☐	☐
☐	☐	☐	☐	☐	☐	☐
☐	☐	☐	☐	☐	☐	☐
☐	☐	☐	☐	☐	☐	☐
☐	☐	☐	☐	☐	☐	☐
☐	☐	☐	☐	☐	☐	☐
☐	☐	☐	☐	☐	☐	☐

QUOTE OF THE DAY

TODAY I AM GRATEFUL FOR:

My Week at a Glance

Week of: ______________

MY WEEKLY AGENDA: NOTES

Sunday ....

Monday ....

Tuesday ....

Wednesday ....

Thursday ....

Friday ....

Saturday ....

TOP GOALS

HEALTHY EATING TRACKER

M	T	W	T	F	S	S
☐	☐	☐	☐	☐	☐	☐
☐	☐	☐	☐	☐	☐	☐
☐	☐	☐	☐	☐	☐	☐
☐	☐	☐	☐	☐	☐	☐
☐	☐	☐	☐	☐	☐	☐
☐	☐	☐	☐	☐	☐	☐
☐	☐	☐	☐	☐	☐	☐
☐	☐	☐	☐	☐	☐	☐

TOP TO DO OF THE WEEK

QUOTE OF THE DAY

TODAY I AM GRATEFUL FOR:

My Week at a Glance

Week of: ____________________

MY WEEKLY AGENDA: NOTES

Sunday ....

Monday ....

Tuesday ....

Wednesday ....

Thursday ....

Friday ....

Saturday ....

TOP GOALS

TOP TO DO OF THE WEEK

HEALTHY EATING TRACKER

M	T	W	T	F	S	S
☐	☐	☐	☐	☐	☐	☐
☐	☐	☐	☐	☐	☐	☐
☐	☐	☐	☐	☐	☐	☐
☐	☐	☐	☐	☐	☐	☐
☐	☐	☐	☐	☐	☐	☐
☐	☐	☐	☐	☐	☐	☐
☐	☐	☐	☐	☐	☐	☐
☐	☐	☐	☐	☐	☐	☐

QUOTE OF THE DAY

TODAY I AM GRATEFUL FOR:

My Week at a Glance

Week of:____________________

MY WEEKLY AGENDA: NOTES

Sunday ....

Monday ....

Tuesday ....

Wednesday ....

Thursday ....

Friday ....

Saturday ....

TOP GOALS

TOP TO DO OF THE WEEK

HEALTHY EATING TRACKER

M	T	W	T	F	S	S
☐	☐	☐	☐	☐	☐	☐
☐	☐	☐	☐	☐	☐	☐
☐	☐	☐	☐	☐	☐	☐
☐	☐	☐	☐	☐	☐	☐
☐	☐	☐	☐	☐	☐	☐
☐	☐	☐	☐	☐	☐	☐
☐	☐	☐	☐	☐	☐	☐
☐	☐	☐	☐	☐	☐	☐

QUOTE OF THE DAY

TODAY I AM GRATEFUL FOR:

My Week at a Glance

Week of: ____________________

MY WEEKLY AGENDA: NOTES

Sunday ....

Monday ....

Tuesday ....

Wednesday ....

Thursday ....

Friday ....

Saturday ....

TOP GOALS

HEALTHY EATING TRACKER

M	T	W	T	F	S	S
☐	☐	☐	☐	☐	☐	☐
☐	☐	☐	☐	☐	☐	☐
☐	☐	☐	☐	☐	☐	☐
☐	☐	☐	☐	☐	☐	☐
☐	☐	☐	☐	☐	☐	☐
☐	☐	☐	☐	☐	☐	☐
☐	☐	☐	☐	☐	☐	☐
☐	☐	☐	☐	☐	☐	☐

TOP TO DO OF THE WEEK

QUOTE OF THE DAY

TODAY I AM GRATEFUL FOR:

My Week at a Glance

Week of: ____________________

MY WEEKLY AGENDA: NOTES

Sunday ....

Monday ....

Tuesday ....

Wednesday ....

Thursday ....

Friday ....

Saturday ....

TOP GOALS

TOP TO DO OF THE WEEK

HEALTHY EATING TRACKER

M	T	W	T	F	S	S
☐	☐	☐	☐	☐	☐	☐
☐	☐	☐	☐	☐	☐	☐
☐	☐	☐	☐	☐	☐	☐
☐	☐	☐	☐	☐	☐	☐
☐	☐	☐	☐	☐	☐	☐
☐	☐	☐	☐	☐	☐	☐
☐	☐	☐	☐	☐	☐	☐
☐	☐	☐	☐	☐	☐	☐

QUOTE OF THE DAY

TODAY I AM GRATEFUL FOR:

My Week at a Glance

Week of: ____________________

MY WEEKLY AGENDA: NOTES

Sunday ....

Monday ....

Tuesday ....

Wednesday ....

Thursday ....

Friday ....

Saturday ....

TOP GOALS

TOP TO DO OF THE WEEK

HEALTHY EATING TRACKER

M	T	W	T	F	S	S

QUOTE OF THE DAY

TODAY I AM GRATEFUL FOR:

My Week at a Glance

Week of: ____________________

MY WEEKLY AGENDA: NOTES

Sunday ....

Monday ....

Tuesday ....

Wednesday ....

Thursday ....

Friday ....

Saturday ....

TOP GOALS

TOP TO DO OF THE WEEK

HEALTHY EATING TRACKER

M	T	W	T	F	S	S

QUOTE OF THE DAY

TODAY I AM GRATEFUL FOR:

My Week at a Glance

Week of: ____________________

MY WEEKLY AGENDA: NOTES

Sunday ....

Monday ....

Tuesday ....

Wednesday ....

Thursday ....

Friday ....

Saturday ....

TOP GOALS

TOP TO DO OF THE WEEK

HEALTHY EATING TRACKER

M	T	W	T	F	S	S
☐	☐	☐	☐	☐	☐	☐
☐	☐	☐	☐	☐	☐	☐
☐	☐	☐	☐	☐	☐	☐
☐	☐	☐	☐	☐	☐	☐
☐	☐	☐	☐	☐	☐	☐
☐	☐	☐	☐	☐	☐	☐
☐	☐	☐	☐	☐	☐	☐
☐	☐	☐	☐	☐	☐	☐

QUOTE OF THE DAY

TODAY I AM GRATEFUL FOR:

My Week at a Glance

Week of:________________

MY WEEKLY AGENDA: NOTES

Sunday ....

Monday ....

Tuesday ....

Wednesday ....

Thursday ....

Friday ....

Saturday ....

TOP GOALS

TOP TO DO OF THE WEEK

HEALTHY EATING TRACKER

M	T	W	T	F	S	S
☐	☐	☐	☐	☐	☐	☐
☐	☐	☐	☐	☐	☐	☐
☐	☐	☐	☐	☐	☐	☐
☐	☐	☐	☐	☐	☐	☐
☐	☐	☐	☐	☐	☐	☐
☐	☐	☐	☐	☐	☐	☐
☐	☐	☐	☐	☐	☐	☐
☐	☐	☐	☐	☐	☐	☐

QUOTE OF THE DAY

TODAY I AM GRATEFUL FOR:

My Week at a Glance

Week of: ____________________

MY WEEKLY AGENDA: NOTES

Sunday ....

Monday ....

Tuesday ....

Wednesday ....

Thursday ....

Friday ....

Saturday ....

TOP GOALS

HEALTHY EATING TRACKER

M	T	W	T	F	S	S
☐	☐	☐	☐	☐	☐	☐
☐	☐	☐	☐	☐	☐	☐
☐	☐	☐	☐	☐	☐	☐
☐	☐	☐	☐	☐	☐	☐
☐	☐	☐	☐	☐	☐	☐
☐	☐	☐	☐	☐	☐	☐
☐	☐	☐	☐	☐	☐	☐
☐	☐	☐	☐	☐	☐	☐

TOP TO DO OF THE WEEK

QUOTE OF THE DAY

TODAY I AM GRATEFUL FOR:

My Week at a Glance

Week of: ____________________

MY WEEKLY AGENDA: NOTES

Sunday ....

Monday ....

Tuesday ....

Wednesday ....

Thursday ....

Friday ....

Saturday ....

TOP GOALS

HEALTHY EATING TRACKER

M	T	W	T	F	S	S
☐	☐	☐	☐	☐	☐	☐
☐	☐	☐	☐	☐	☐	☐
☐	☐	☐	☐	☐	☐	☐
☐	☐	☐	☐	☐	☐	☐
☐	☐	☐	☐	☐	☐	☐
☐	☐	☐	☐	☐	☐	☐
☐	☐	☐	☐	☐	☐	☐
☐	☐	☐	☐	☐	☐	☐

TOP TO DO OF THE WEEK

QUOTE OF THE DAY

TODAY I AM GRATEFUL FOR:

My Week at a Glance

Week of: ____________________

MY WEEKLY AGENDA: NOTES

Sunday ....

Monday ....

Tuesday ....

Wednesday ....

Thursday ....

Friday ....

Saturday ....

TOP GOALS

TOP TO DO OF THE WEEK

HEALTHY EATING TRACKER

M	T	W	T	F	S	S
☐	☐	☐	☐	☐	☐	☐
☐	☐	☐	☐	☐	☐	☐
☐	☐	☐	☐	☐	☐	☐
☐	☐	☐	☐	☐	☐	☐
☐	☐	☐	☐	☐	☐	☐
☐	☐	☐	☐	☐	☐	☐
☐	☐	☐	☐	☐	☐	☐
☐	☐	☐	☐	☐	☐	☐

QUOTE OF THE DAY

TODAY I AM GRATEFUL FOR:

My Week at a Glance

Week of: ________________

MY WEEKLY AGENDA: NOTES

Sunday ....

Monday ....

Tuesday ....

Wednesday ....

Thursday ....

Friday ....

Saturday ....

TOP GOALS

TOP TO DO OF THE WEEK

HEALTHY EATING TRACKER

M	T	W	T	F	S	S
☐	☐	☐	☐	☐	☐	☐
☐	☐	☐	☐	☐	☐	☐
☐	☐	☐	☐	☐	☐	☐
☐	☐	☐	☐	☐	☐	☐
☐	☐	☐	☐	☐	☐	☐
☐	☐	☐	☐	☐	☐	☐
☐	☐	☐	☐	☐	☐	☐
☐	☐	☐	☐	☐	☐	☐

QUOTE OF THE DAY

TODAY I AM GRATEFUL FOR:

My Week at a Glance

Week of: ____________________

MY WEEKLY AGENDA: NOTES

Sunday ....

Monday ....

Tuesday ....

Wednesday ....

Thursday ....

Friday ....

Saturday ....

TOP GOALS

HEALTHY EATING TRACKER

M	T	W	T	F	S	S
☐	☐	☐	☐	☐	☐	☐
☐	☐	☐	☐	☐	☐	☐
☐	☐	☐	☐	☐	☐	☐
☐	☐	☐	☐	☐	☐	☐
☐	☐	☐	☐	☐	☐	☐
☐	☐	☐	☐	☐	☐	☐
☐	☐	☐	☐	☐	☐	☐
☐	☐	☐	☐	☐	☐	☐

TOP TO DO OF THE WEEK

QUOTE OF THE DAY

TODAY I AM GRATEFUL FOR:

My Week at a Glance

Week of: ____________________

MY WEEKLY AGENDA: NOTES

Sunday ....

Monday ....

Tuesday ....

Wednesday ....

Thursday ....

Friday ....

Saturday ....

TOP GOALS

TOP TO DO OF THE WEEK

HEALTHY EATING TRACKER

M	T	W	T	F	S	S
☐	☐	☐	☐	☐	☐	☐
☐	☐	☐	☐	☐	☐	☐
☐	☐	☐	☐	☐	☐	☐
☐	☐	☐	☐	☐	☐	☐
☐	☐	☐	☐	☐	☐	☐
☐	☐	☐	☐	☐	☐	☐
☐	☐	☐	☐	☐	☐	☐
☐	☐	☐	☐	☐	☐	☐

QUOTE OF THE DAY

TODAY I AM GRATEFUL FOR:

My Week at a Glance

Week of: ____________________

MY WEEKLY AGENDA: NOTES

Sunday ....

Monday ....

Tuesday ....

Wednesday ....

Thursday ....

Friday ....

Saturday ....

TOP GOALS

TOP TO DO OF THE WEEK

HEALTHY EATING TRACKER

M	T	W	T	F	S	S
☐	☐	☐	☐	☐	☐	☐
☐	☐	☐	☐	☐	☐	☐
☐	☐	☐	☐	☐	☐	☐
☐	☐	☐	☐	☐	☐	☐
☐	☐	☐	☐	☐	☐	☐
☐	☐	☐	☐	☐	☐	☐
☐	☐	☐	☐	☐	☐	☐
☐	☐	☐	☐	☐	☐	☐

QUOTE OF THE DAY

TODAY I AM GRATEFUL FOR:

My Week at a Glance

Week of: ____________________

MY WEEKLY AGENDA: NOTES

Sunday ....

Monday ....

Tuesday ....

Wednesday ....

Thursday ....

Friday ....

Saturday ....

TOP GOALS

HEALTHY EATING TRACKER

M	T	W	T	F	S	S
☐	☐	☐	☐	☐	☐	☐
☐	☐	☐	☐	☐	☐	☐
☐	☐	☐	☐	☐	☐	☐
☐	☐	☐	☐	☐	☐	☐
☐	☐	☐	☐	☐	☐	☐
☐	☐	☐	☐	☐	☐	☐
☐	☐	☐	☐	☐	☐	☐
☐	☐	☐	☐	☐	☐	☐

TOP TO DO OF THE WEEK

QUOTE OF THE DAY

TODAY I AM GRATEFUL FOR:

My Week at a Glance

Week of: ____________

MY WEEKLY AGENDA: NOTES

Sunday ....

Monday ....

Tuesday ....

Wednesday ....

Thursday ....

Friday ....

Saturday ....

TOP GOALS

TOP TO DO OF THE WEEK

HEALTHY EATING TRACKER

M	T	W	T	F	S	S
☐	☐	☐	☐	☐	☐	☐
☐	☐	☐	☐	☐	☐	☐
☐	☐	☐	☐	☐	☐	☐
☐	☐	☐	☐	☐	☐	☐
☐	☐	☐	☐	☐	☐	☐
☐	☐	☐	☐	☐	☐	☐
☐	☐	☐	☐	☐	☐	☐
☐	☐	☐	☐	☐	☐	☐

QUOTE OF THE DAY

TODAY I AM GRATEFUL FOR:

My Week at a Glance

Week of:____________________

MY WEEKLY AGENDA: NOTES

Sunday ....

Monday ....

Tuesday ....

Wednesday ....

Thursday ....

Friday ....

Saturday ....

TOP GOALS

TOP TO DO OF THE WEEK

HEALTHY EATING TRACKER

M	T	W	T	F	S	S
☐	☐	☐	☐	☐	☐	☐
☐	☐	☐	☐	☐	☐	☐
☐	☐	☐	☐	☐	☐	☐
☐	☐	☐	☐	☐	☐	☐
☐	☐	☐	☐	☐	☐	☐
☐	☐	☐	☐	☐	☐	☐
☐	☐	☐	☐	☐	☐	☐
☐	☐	☐	☐	☐	☐	☐

QUOTE OF THE DAY

TODAY I AM GRATEFUL FOR:

My Week at a Glance

Week of: ____________________

MY WEEKLY AGENDA: NOTES

Sunday ....

Monday ....

Tuesday ....

Wednesday ....

Thursday ....

Friday ....

Saturday ....

TOP GOALS

TOP TO DO OF THE WEEK

HEALTHY EATING TRACKER

M	T	W	T	F	S	S
☐	☐	☐	☐	☐	☐	☐
☐	☐	☐	☐	☐	☐	☐
☐	☐	☐	☐	☐	☐	☐
☐	☐	☐	☐	☐	☐	☐
☐	☐	☐	☐	☐	☐	☐
☐	☐	☐	☐	☐	☐	☐
☐	☐	☐	☐	☐	☐	☐
☐	☐	☐	☐	☐	☐	☐

QUOTE OF THE DAY

TODAY I AM GRATEFUL FOR:

My Week at a Glance

Week of: ____________________

MY WEEKLY AGENDA: NOTES
Sunday ....
Monday ....
Tuesday ....
Wednesday ....
Thursday ....
Friday ....
Saturday ....

TOP GOALS

HEALTHY EATING TRACKER

M	T	W	T	F	S	S
☐	☐	☐	☐	☐	☐	☐
☐	☐	☐	☐	☐	☐	☐
☐	☐	☐	☐	☐	☐	☐
☐	☐	☐	☐	☐	☐	☐
☐	☐	☐	☐	☐	☐	☐
☐	☐	☐	☐	☐	☐	☐
☐	☐	☐	☐	☐	☐	☐
☐	☐	☐	☐	☐	☐	☐

TOP TO DO OF THE WEEK

QUOTE OF THE DAY

TODAY I AM GRATEFUL FOR:

My Week at a Glance

Week of: ____________

MY WEEKLY AGENDA: NOTES

Sunday ....

Monday ....

Tuesday ....

Wednesday ....

Thursday ....

Friday ....

Saturday ....

TOP GOALS

TOP TO DO OF THE WEEK

HEALTHY EATING TRACKER

M	T	W	T	F	S	S

QUOTE OF THE DAY

TODAY I AM GRATEFUL FOR:

My Week at a Glance

Week of: ____________________

MY WEEKLY AGENDA: NOTES

Sunday ....

Monday ....

Tuesday ....

Wednesday ....

Thursday ....

Friday ....

Saturday ....

TOP GOALS

TOP TO DO OF THE WEEK

HEALTHY EATING TRACKER

M	T	W	T	F	S	S
☐	☐	☐	☐	☐	☐	☐
☐	☐	☐	☐	☐	☐	☐
☐	☐	☐	☐	☐	☐	☐
☐	☐	☐	☐	☐	☐	☐
☐	☐	☐	☐	☐	☐	☐
☐	☐	☐	☐	☐	☐	☐
☐	☐	☐	☐	☐	☐	☐
☐	☐	☐	☐	☐	☐	☐

QUOTE OF THE DAY

TODAY I AM GRATEFUL FOR:

My Week at a Glance

Week of:__________________

MY WEEKLY AGENDA: NOTES

Sunday ....

Monday ....

Tuesday ....

Wednesday ....

Thursday ....

Friday ....

Saturday ....

TOP GOALS

TOP TO DO OF THE WEEK

HEALTHY EATING TRACKER

M	T	W	T	F	S	S
☐	☐	☐	☐	☐	☐	☐
☐	☐	☐	☐	☐	☐	☐
☐	☐	☐	☐	☐	☐	☐
☐	☐	☐	☐	☐	☐	☐
☐	☐	☐	☐	☐	☐	☐
☐	☐	☐	☐	☐	☐	☐
☐	☐	☐	☐	☐	☐	☐
☐	☐	☐	☐	☐	☐	☐

QUOTE OF THE DAY

TODAY I AM GRATEFUL FOR:

My Week at a Glance

Week of: ____________

MY WEEKLY AGENDA: NOTES

Sunday ....

Monday ....

Tuesday ....

Wednesday ....

Thursday ....

Friday ....

Saturday ....

TOP GOALS

HEALTHY EATING TRACKER

M	T	W	T	F	S	S
☐	☐	☐	☐	☐	☐	☐
☐	☐	☐	☐	☐	☐	☐
☐	☐	☐	☐	☐	☐	☐
☐	☐	☐	☐	☐	☐	☐
☐	☐	☐	☐	☐	☐	☐
☐	☐	☐	☐	☐	☐	☐
☐	☐	☐	☐	☐	☐	☐
☐	☐	☐	☐	☐	☐	☐

TOP TO DO OF THE WEEK

QUOTE OF THE DAY

TODAY I AM GRATEFUL FOR:

My Week at a Glance

Week of: ____________________

MY WEEKLY AGENDA: NOTES

Sunday ....

Monday ....

Tuesday ....

Wednesday ....

Thursday ....

Friday ....

Saturday ....

TOP GOALS

TOP TO DO OF THE WEEK

HEALTHY EATING TRACKER

M	T	W	T	F	S	S
☐	☐	☐	☐	☐	☐	☐
☐	☐	☐	☐	☐	☐	☐
☐	☐	☐	☐	☐	☐	☐
☐	☐	☐	☐	☐	☐	☐
☐	☐	☐	☐	☐	☐	☐
☐	☐	☐	☐	☐	☐	☐
☐	☐	☐	☐	☐	☐	☐
☐	☐	☐	☐	☐	☐	☐

QUOTE OF THE DAY

TODAY I AM GRATEFUL FOR:

My Week at a Glance

Week of: ____________________

MY WEEKLY AGENDA: NOTES

Sunday ....

Monday ....

Tuesday ....

Wednesday ....

Thursday ....

Friday ....

Saturday ....

TOP GOALS

TOP TO DO OF THE WEEK

HEALTHY EATING TRACKER

M	T	W	T	F	S	S
☐	☐	☐	☐	☐	☐	☐
☐	☐	☐	☐	☐	☐	☐
☐	☐	☐	☐	☐	☐	☐
☐	☐	☐	☐	☐	☐	☐
☐	☐	☐	☐	☐	☐	☐
☐	☐	☐	☐	☐	☐	☐
☐	☐	☐	☐	☐	☐	☐
☐	☐	☐	☐	☐	☐	☐

QUOTE OF THE DAY

TODAY I AM GRATEFUL FOR:

My Week at a Glance

Week of: ______________________

MY WEEKLY AGENDA: NOTES

Sunday ....

Monday ....

Tuesday ....

Wednesday ....

Thursday ....

Friday ....

Saturday ....

TOP GOALS

TOP TO DO OF THE WEEK

HEALTHY EATING TRACKER

M	T	W	T	F	S	S

QUOTE OF THE DAY

TODAY I AM GRATEFUL FOR:

My Week at a Glance

Week of: ____________

MY WEEKLY AGENDA: NOTES

Sunday ....

Monday ....

Tuesday ....

Wednesday ....

Thursday ....

Friday ....

Saturday ....

TOP GOALS

TOP TO DO OF THE WEEK

HEALTHY EATING TRACKER

M	T	W	T	F	S	S
☐	☐	☐	☐	☐	☐	☐
☐	☐	☐	☐	☐	☐	☐
☐	☐	☐	☐	☐	☐	☐
☐	☐	☐	☐	☐	☐	☐
☐	☐	☐	☐	☐	☐	☐
☐	☐	☐	☐	☐	☐	☐
☐	☐	☐	☐	☐	☐	☐
☐	☐	☐	☐	☐	☐	☐

QUOTE OF THE DAY

TODAY I AM GRATEFUL FOR:

My Week at a Glance

Week of: ____________________

MY WEEKLY AGENDA: NOTES

Sunday ....

Monday ....

Tuesday ....

Wednesday ....

Thursday ....

Friday ....

Saturday ....

TOP GOALS

TOP TO DO OF THE WEEK

HEALTHY EATING TRACKER

M	T	W	T	F	S	S
☐	☐	☐	☐	☐	☐	☐
☐	☐	☐	☐	☐	☐	☐
☐	☐	☐	☐	☐	☐	☐
☐	☐	☐	☐	☐	☐	☐
☐	☐	☐	☐	☐	☐	☐
☐	☐	☐	☐	☐	☐	☐
☐	☐	☐	☐	☐	☐	☐
☐	☐	☐	☐	☐	☐	☐

QUOTE OF THE DAY

TODAY I AM GRATEFUL FOR:

My Week at a Glance

Week of: ______________

MY WEEKLY AGENDA: NOTES

Sunday ....

Monday ....

Tuesday ....

Wednesday ....

Thursday ....

Friday ....

Saturday ....

TOP GOALS

TOP TO DO OF THE WEEK

HEALTHY EATING TRACKER

M	T	W	T	F	S	S
☐	☐	☐	☐	☐	☐	☐
☐	☐	☐	☐	☐	☐	☐
☐	☐	☐	☐	☐	☐	☐
☐	☐	☐	☐	☐	☐	☐
☐	☐	☐	☐	☐	☐	☐
☐	☐	☐	☐	☐	☐	☐
☐	☐	☐	☐	☐	☐	☐
☐	☐	☐	☐	☐	☐	☐

QUOTE OF THE DAY

TODAY I AM GRATEFUL FOR:

My Week at a Glance

Week of: ____________________

MY WEEKLY AGENDA: NOTES

Sunday ....

Monday ....

Tuesday ....

Wednesday ....

Thursday ....

Friday ....

Saturday ....

TOP GOALS

TOP TO DO OF THE WEEK

HEALTHY EATING TRACKER

M	T	W	T	F	S	S
☐	☐	☐	☐	☐	☐	☐
☐	☐	☐	☐	☐	☐	☐
☐	☐	☐	☐	☐	☐	☐
☐	☐	☐	☐	☐	☐	☐
☐	☐	☐	☐	☐	☐	☐
☐	☐	☐	☐	☐	☐	☐
☐	☐	☐	☐	☐	☐	☐
☐	☐	☐	☐	☐	☐	☐

QUOTE OF THE DAY

TODAY I AM GRATEFUL FOR:

My Week at a Glance

Week of:________________

MY WEEKLY AGENDA: NOTES

Sunday ....

Monday ....

Tuesday ....

Wednesday ....

Thursday ....

Friday ....

Saturday ....

TOP GOALS

TOP TO DO OF THE WEEK

HEALTHY EATING TRACKER

M	T	W	T	F	S	S
☐	☐	☐	☐	☐	☐	☐
☐	☐	☐	☐	☐	☐	☐
☐	☐	☐	☐	☐	☐	☐
☐	☐	☐	☐	☐	☐	☐
☐	☐	☐	☐	☐	☐	☐
☐	☐	☐	☐	☐	☐	☐
☐	☐	☐	☐	☐	☐	☐
☐	☐	☐	☐	☐	☐	☐

QUOTE OF THE DAY

TODAY I AM GRATEFUL FOR:

My Week at a Glance

Week of: ____________________

MY WEEKLY AGENDA: NOTES

Sunday ....

Monday ....

Tuesday ....

Wednesday ....

Thursday ....

Friday ....

Saturday ....

TOP GOALS

TOP TO DO OF THE WEEK

HEALTHY EATING TRACKER

M	T	W	T	F	S	S
☐	☐	☐	☐	☐	☐	☐
☐	☐	☐	☐	☐	☐	☐
☐	☐	☐	☐	☐	☐	☐
☐	☐	☐	☐	☐	☐	☐
☐	☐	☐	☐	☐	☐	☐
☐	☐	☐	☐	☐	☐	☐
☐	☐	☐	☐	☐	☐	☐
☐	☐	☐	☐	☐	☐	☐

QUOTE OF THE DAY

TODAY I AM GRATEFUL FOR:

My Week at a Glance

Week of: ____________

MY WEEKLY AGENDA: NOTES

Sunday ....

Monday ....

Tuesday ....

Wednesday ....

Thursday ....

Friday ....

Saturday ....

TOP GOALS

TOP TO DO OF THE WEEK

HEALTHY EATING TRACKER

M	T	W	T	F	S	S
☐	☐	☐	☐	☐	☐	☐
☐	☐	☐	☐	☐	☐	☐
☐	☐	☐	☐	☐	☐	☐
☐	☐	☐	☐	☐	☐	☐
☐	☐	☐	☐	☐	☐	☐
☐	☐	☐	☐	☐	☐	☐
☐	☐	☐	☐	☐	☐	☐
☐	☐	☐	☐	☐	☐	☐

QUOTE OF THE DAY

TODAY I AM GRATEFUL FOR:

My Week at a Glance

Week of: ____________

MY WEEKLY AGENDA: NOTES

Sunday ....

Monday ....

Tuesday ....

Wednesday ....

Thursday ....

Friday ....

Saturday ....

TOP GOALS

HEALTHY EATING TRACKER

M	T	W	T	F	S	S

TOP TO DO OF THE WEEK

QUOTE OF THE DAY

TODAY I AM GRATEFUL FOR:

My Week at a Glance

Week of: ____________________

MY WEEKLY AGENDA: NOTES

Sunday ....

Monday ....

Tuesday ....

Wednesday ....

Thursday ....

Friday ....

Saturday ....

TOP GOALS

HEALTHY EATING TRACKER

M	T	W	T	F	S	S
☐	☐	☐	☐	☐	☐	☐
☐	☐	☐	☐	☐	☐	☐
☐	☐	☐	☐	☐	☐	☐
☐	☐	☐	☐	☐	☐	☐
☐	☐	☐	☐	☐	☐	☐
☐	☐	☐	☐	☐	☐	☐
☐	☐	☐	☐	☐	☐	☐
☐	☐	☐	☐	☐	☐	☐

TOP TO DO OF THE WEEK

QUOTE OF THE DAY

TODAY I AM GRATEFUL FOR:

Notes and Things

Coloring Pages

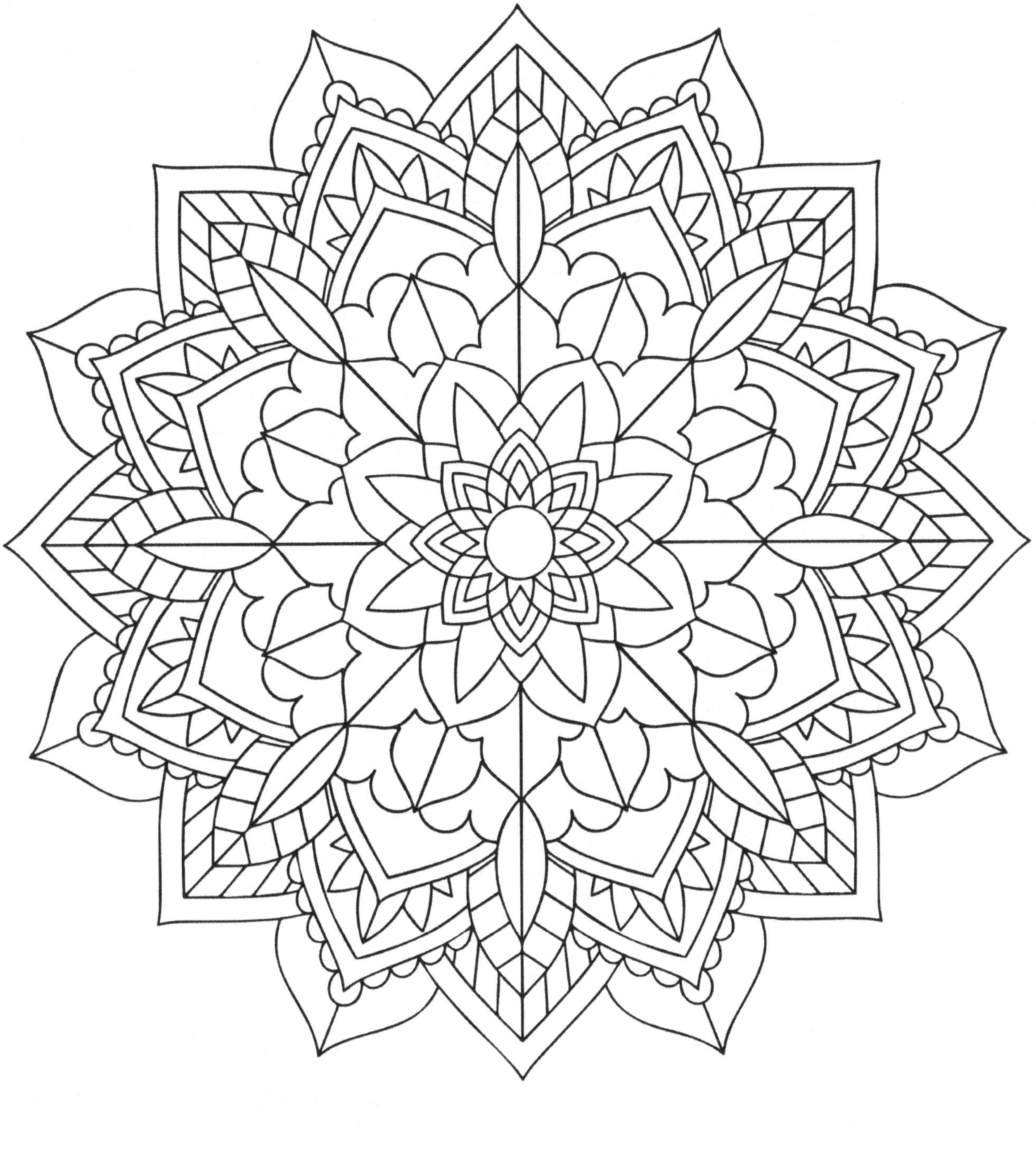

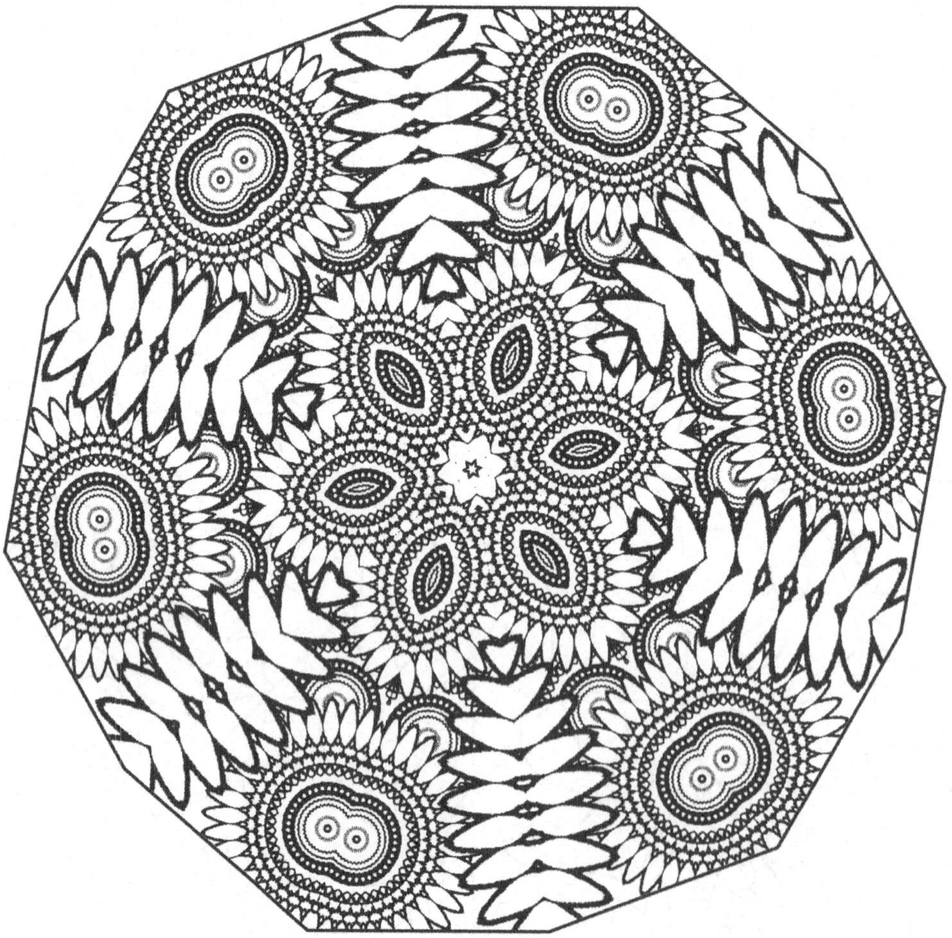

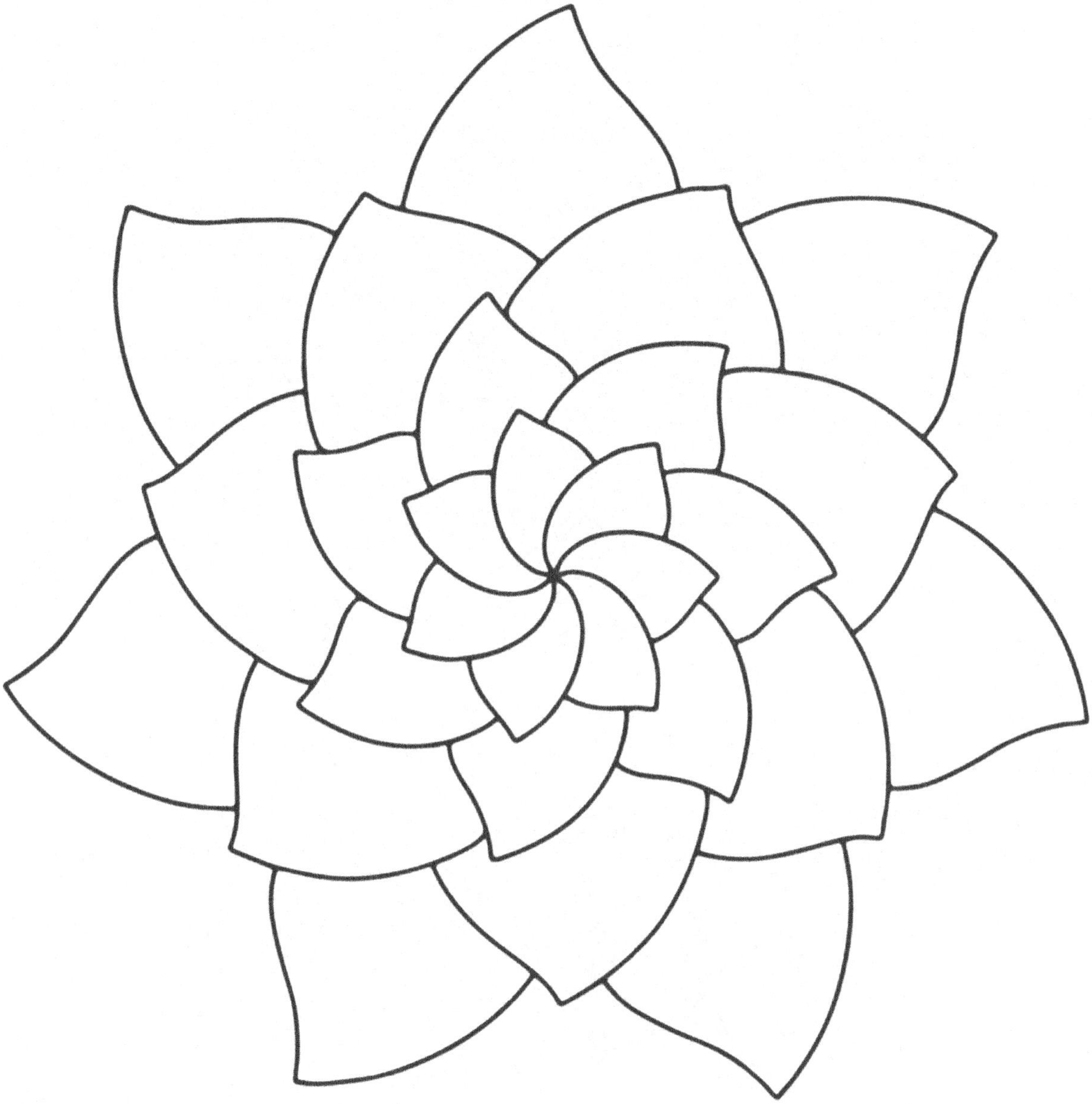

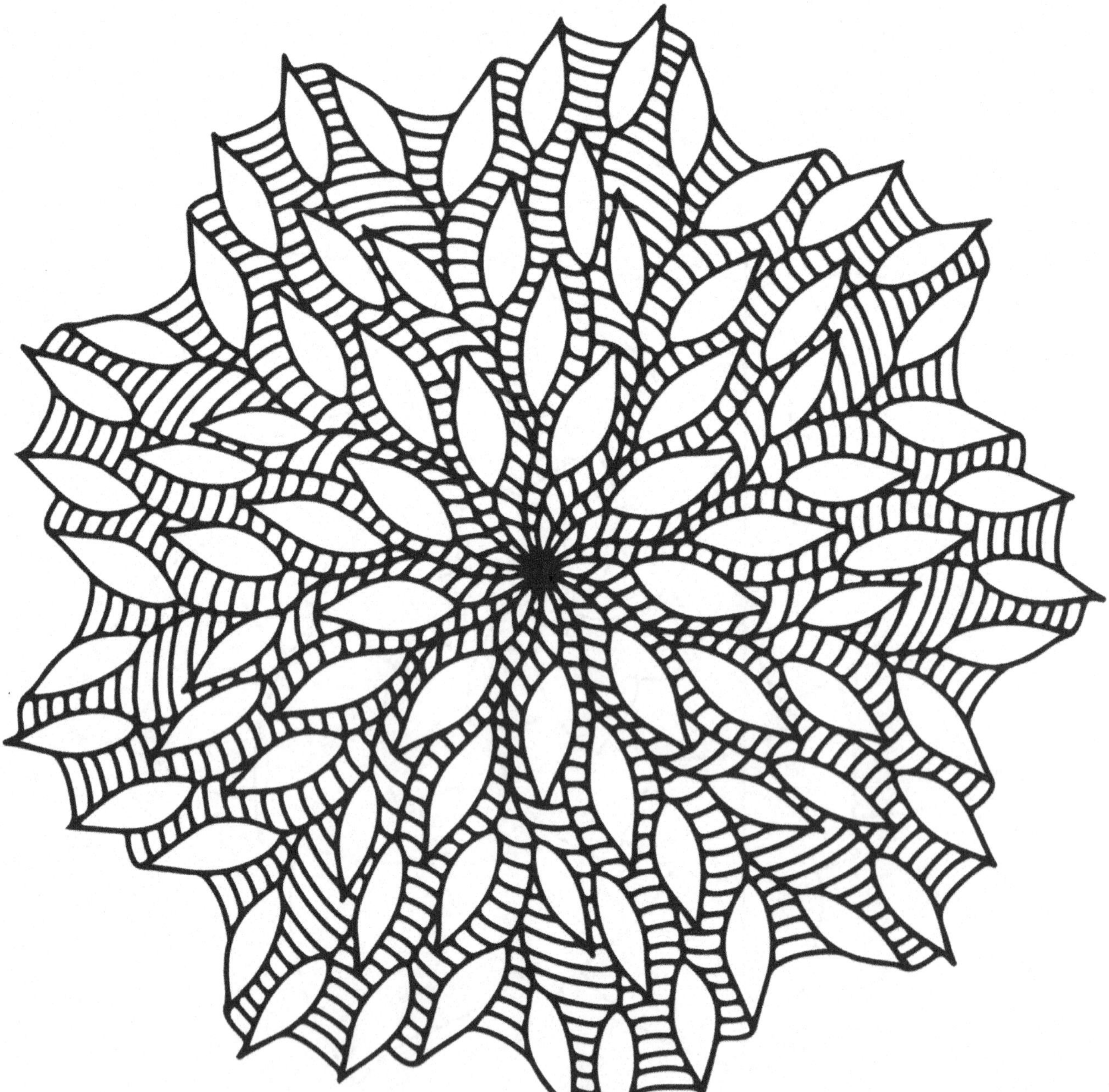

Made in the USA
Columbia, SC
17 September 2020

20930126R00050